Large Print

Stroke Warriors

Cognitive Comeback

Brain Injury and
Global Aphasia Rehabilitation
Activity Book

Solution Included

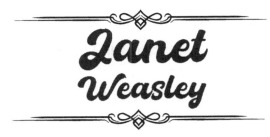

Janet
Weasley

This book belongs to

Table of Contents

Good Luck

We want to commend you on taking the initiative to purchase the "Stroke Recovery Activity Book." This book is an excellent choice that will greatly support your journey towards stroke recovery.

The **"Stroke Recovery Activity Book"** offers a comprehensive range of exercises and tasks that cater to various aspects of rehabilitation. The activities within this book have been carefully crafted by experts in the field of stroke recovery, ensuring that they are both effective and enjoyable.

Remember, stroke recovery is a journey, and this book will serve as a trusted companion, guiding you towards a brighter future.

Congratulations on your commitment to your recovery, and we wish you every success as you embark on this transformative process.

Warm regards,

Janet
Weasley

Chapter 1
Tracing Trails
Exploring the Path to Stroke Recovery

Trace the Lines

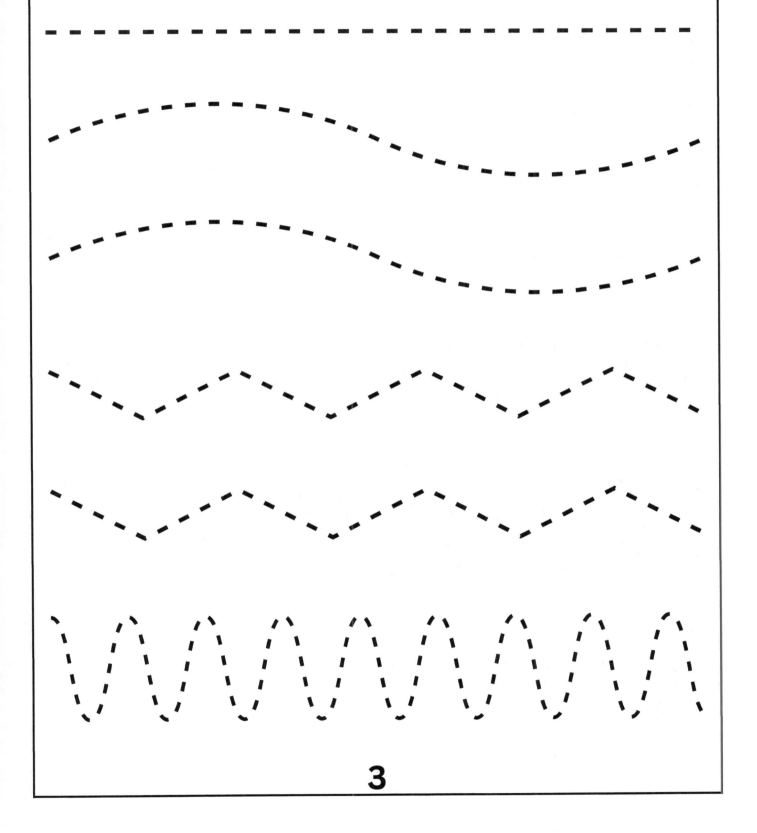

Trace the Lines Given Below.

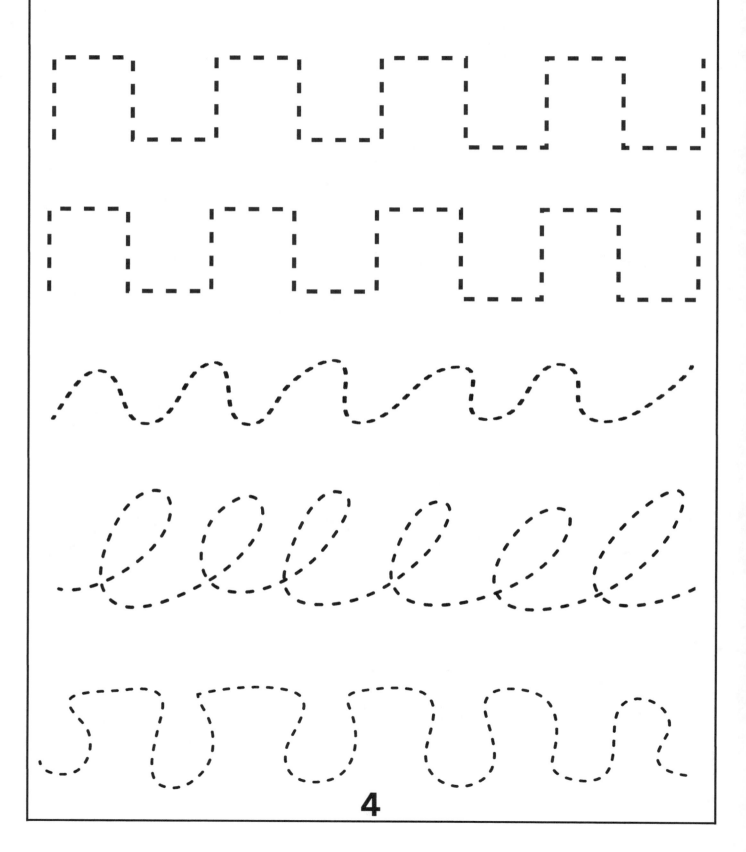

4

Trace the Path and Go to the Fruits.

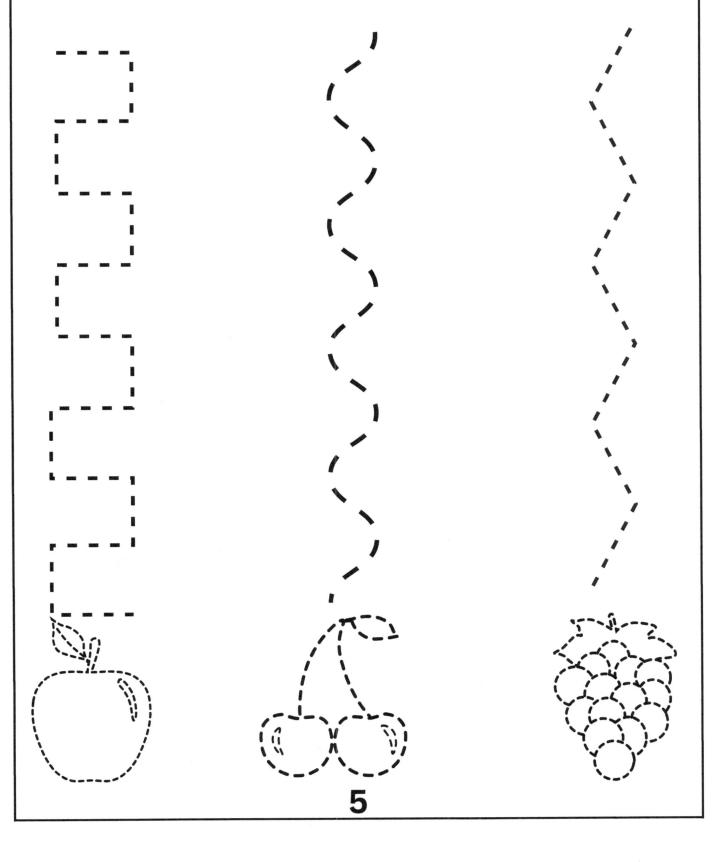

5

Trace the Curves

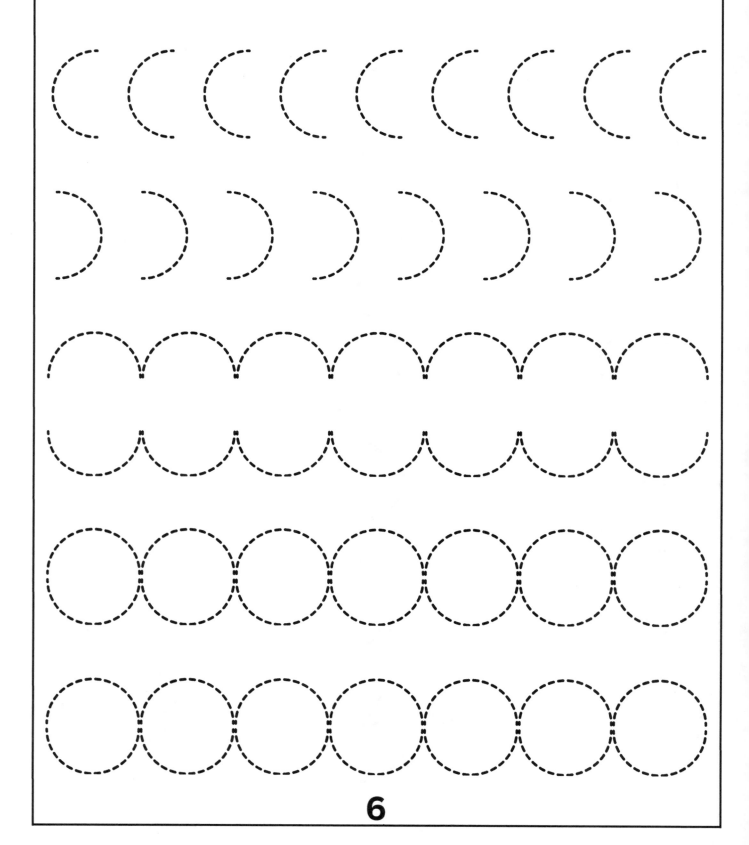

6

Trace the Lines

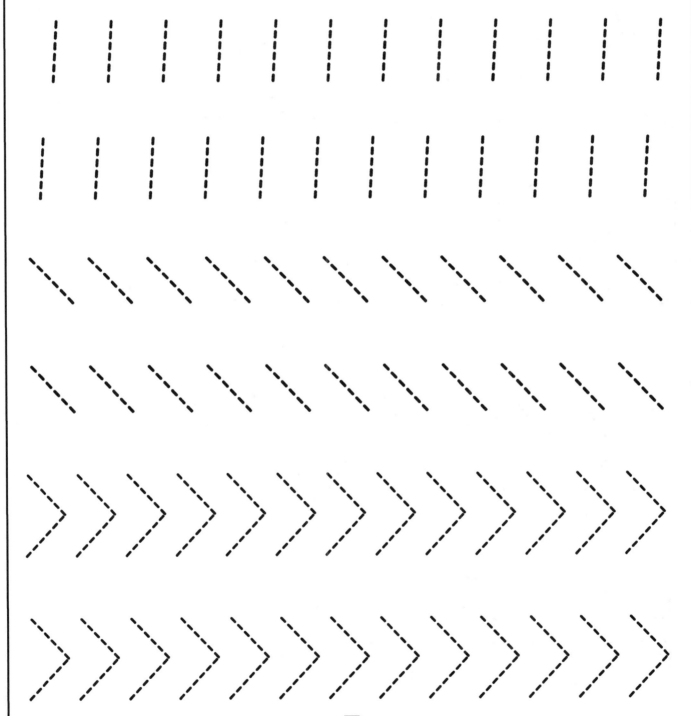

Trace the Patterns

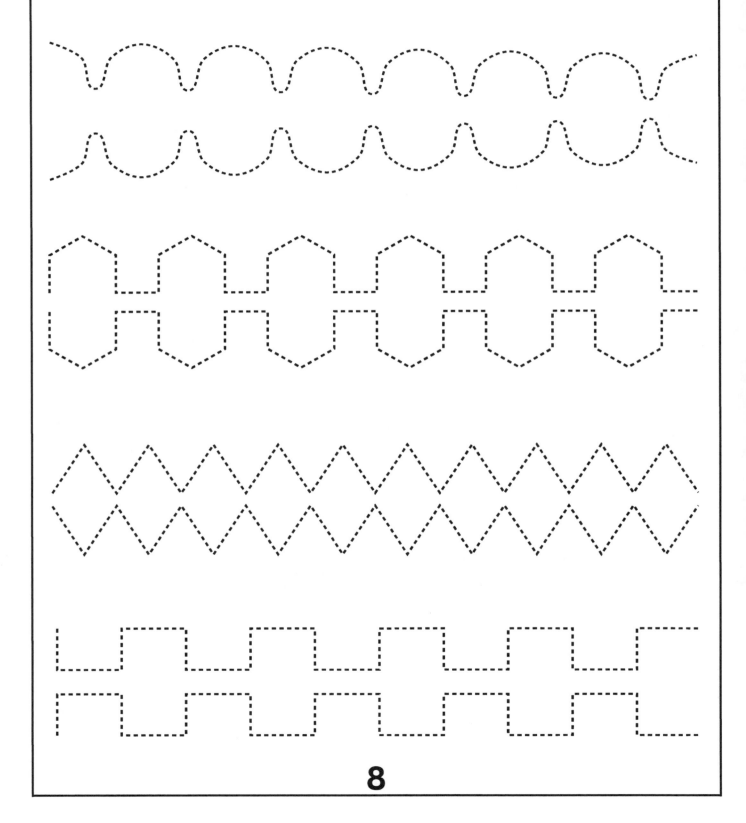

8

Trace and Color the House.

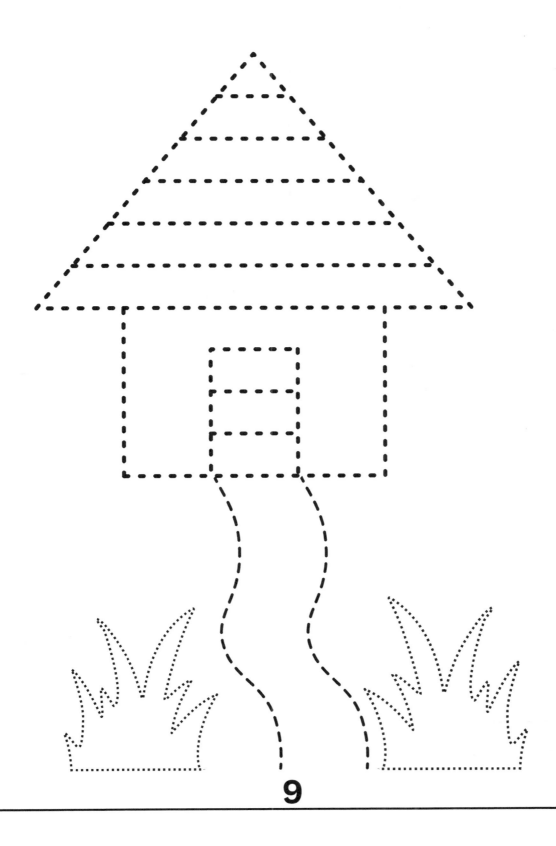

9

Trace and Speak the Name of Each shape

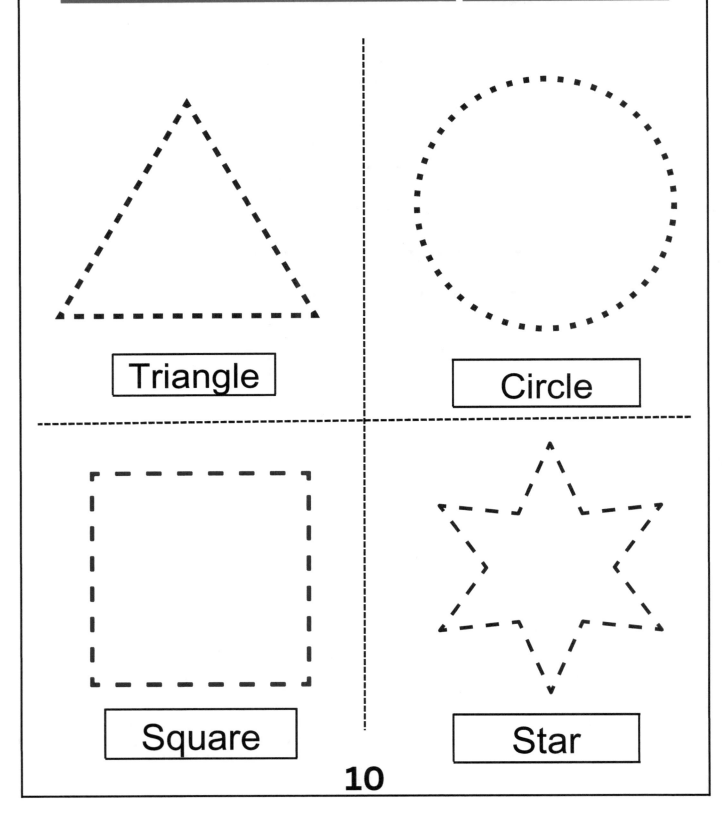

Triangle

Circle

Square

Star

10

Trace and Color the Images

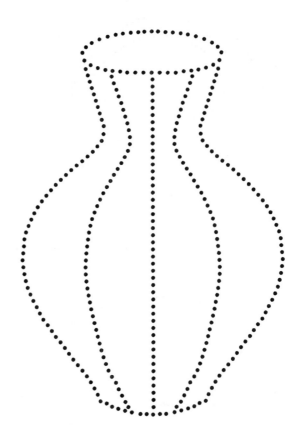

Trace and Draw the Images

Trace	Draw your own

Number Tracing from (1-5)

2 3 4 5

2 3 4 5

2 3 4 5

Number Tracing from(6-10)

6 7 8 9 10

6 7 8 9 10

6 7 8 9 10

13

Letter Tracing from (Aa-Dd)

Aa   Bb   Cc   Dd

Aa   Bb   Cc   Dd

Aa   Bb   Cc   Dd

Letter Tracing from (Ee-Hh)

Ee   Ff   Gg   Hh

Ee   Ff   Gg   Hh

Ee   Ff   Gg   Hh

Letter Tracing from (Ii-Ll)

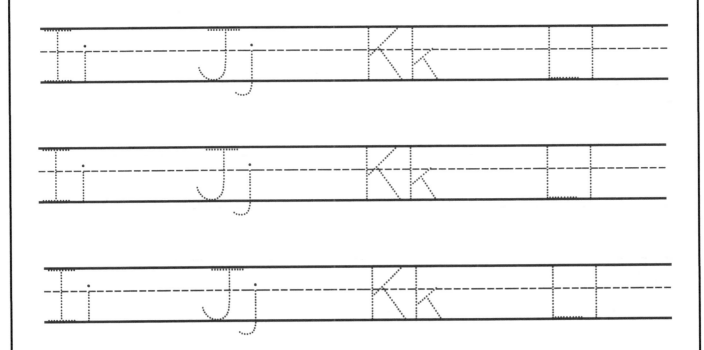

Letter tracing from (Mm-Pp)

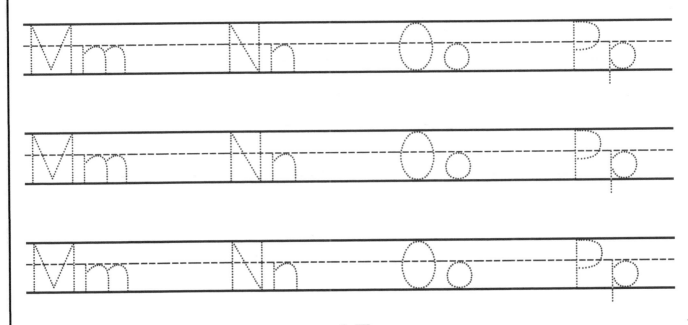

Letter Tracing from (Qq-Tt)

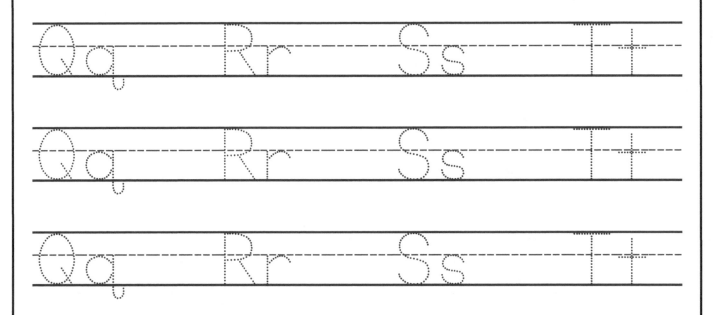

Letter Tracing from (Uu-Xx)

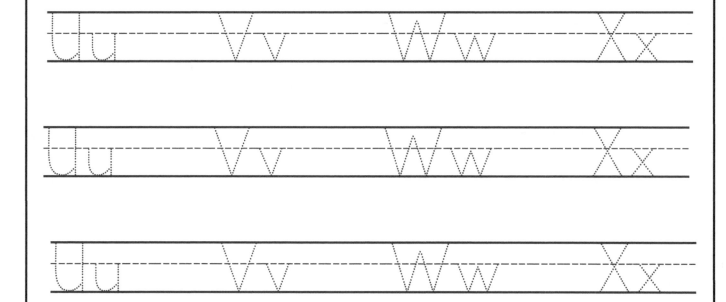

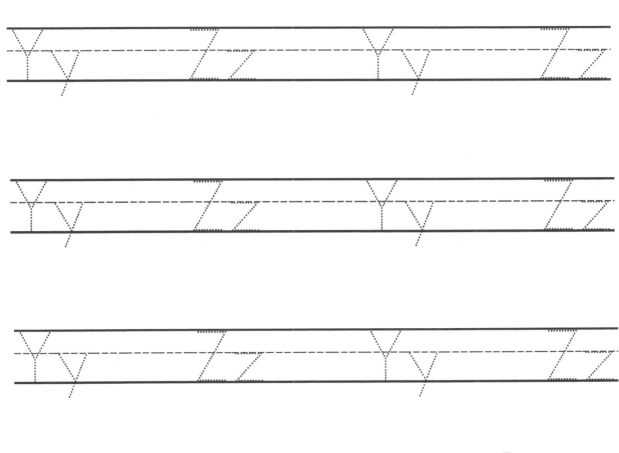

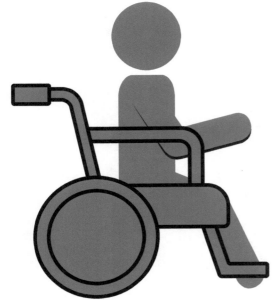

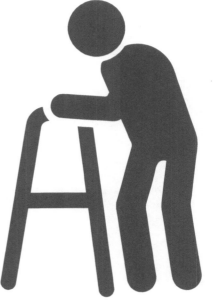

Time for Hand Movement

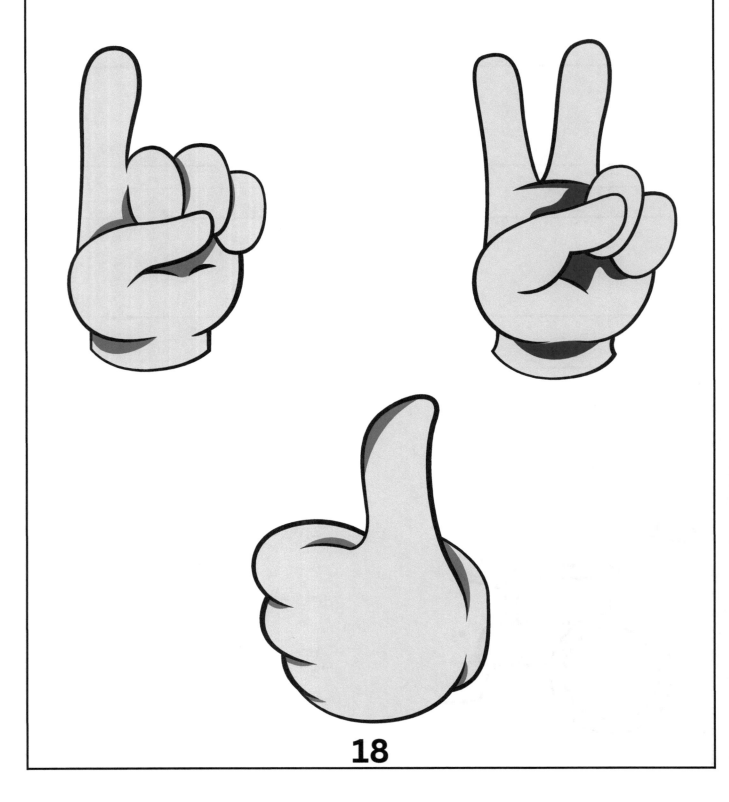

Time for Hand Movement

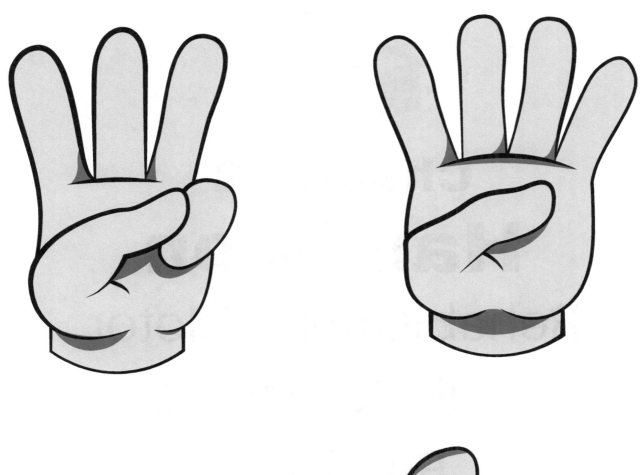

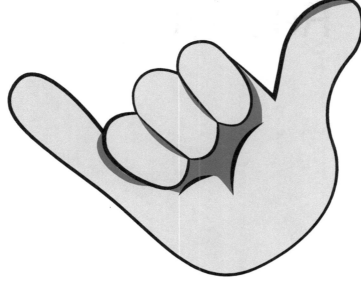

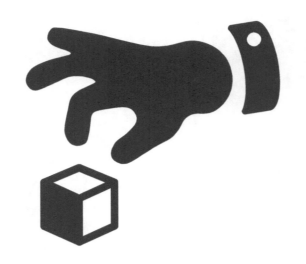

Chapter:2
Hands on
Rehabilitating Motor Skills for Stroke Recovery

Cut and Glue on the Correct Place

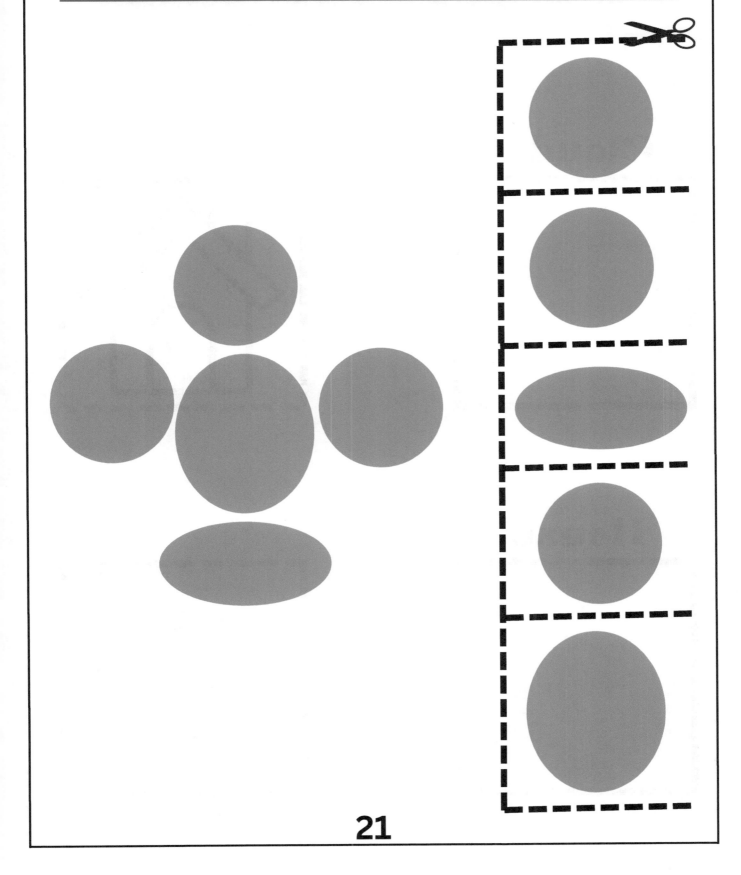

Cut and Glue the Pictures Under the Correct Word.

Cloud

House

22

Draw a Square around the Fruits.

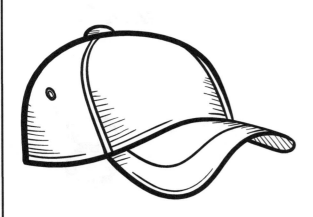

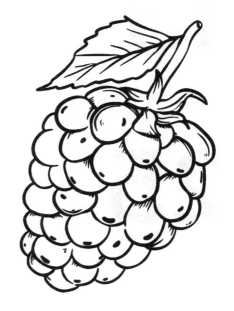

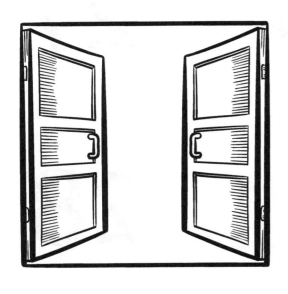

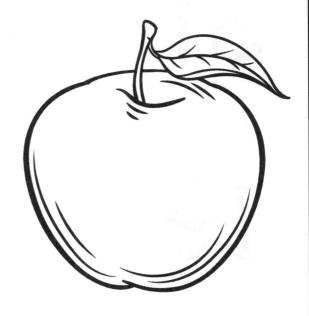

23

Circle the Odd One

13   17   23

25   C   3

31   40   27

19   8   28

Circle the Odd One

r　t　p　s

b　c　l　z

h　n　5　u

x　t　p　y

Letter Hunt

Find all the letters 'x' and circle them.

X   X   Z   U

X   T   (X)   M   X

P   X   W   N

S   X   M   X

Cut and Paste in the Correct Box.

Circle	Rectangle

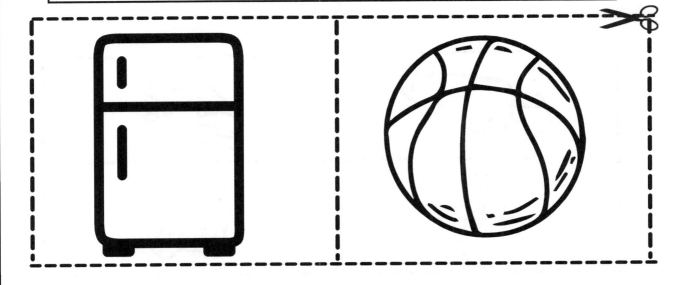

Cut the Picture and Paste Inside Likes or Dislike Sides.

Likes	Dislikes

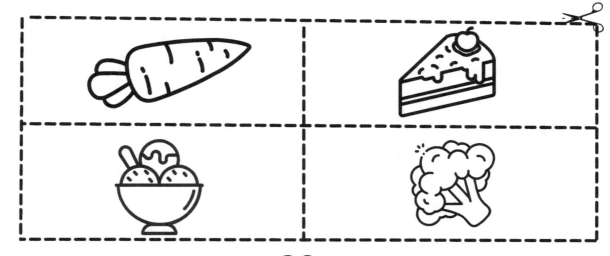

Number Hunt 🔍

Find all the numbers 3 and circle them.

1   3   8   3

3   2   3   4

9   (3)   9

3   5   3   1

7   3   9   3

Trace the Word that does not belong to Each Group.

goat

cow

crow →

----

dog

cat

parrot →

30

Complete the Patterns

Cut and paste the shapes from the boxes below

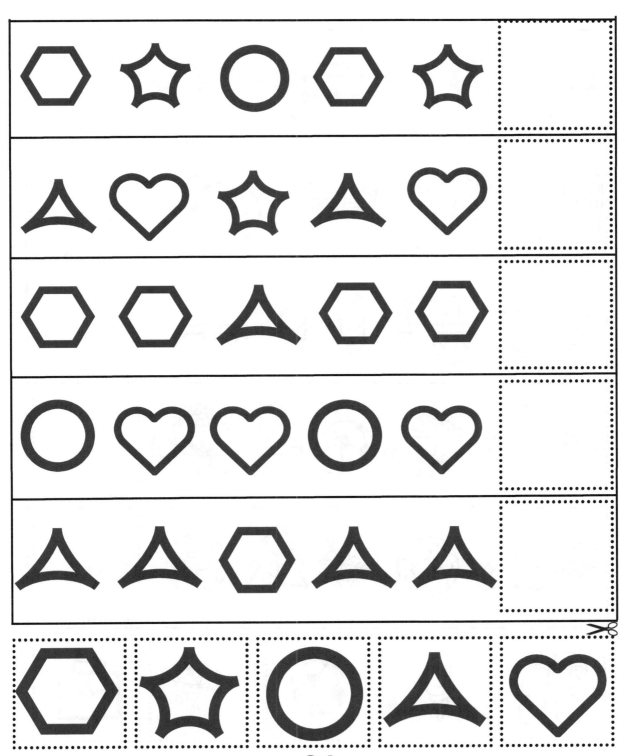

Complete the each Pattern.
Cut and Glue

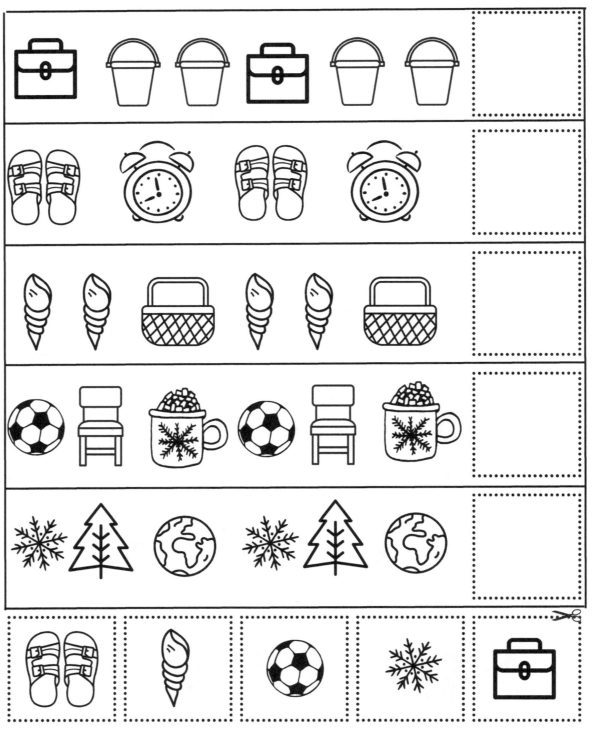

32

Handwriting Practice

Try to write your name and age.

My name is . . . .

I am . . . . years old.

Time for Hand Movement

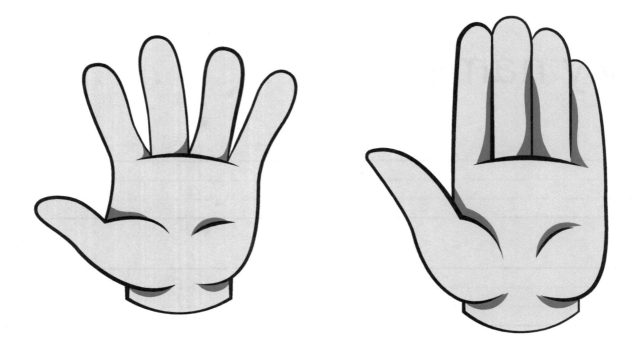

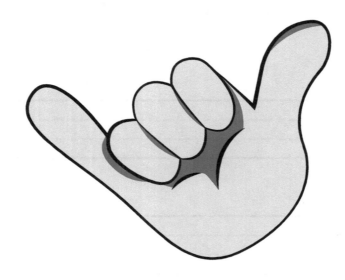

Time for Hand Movement

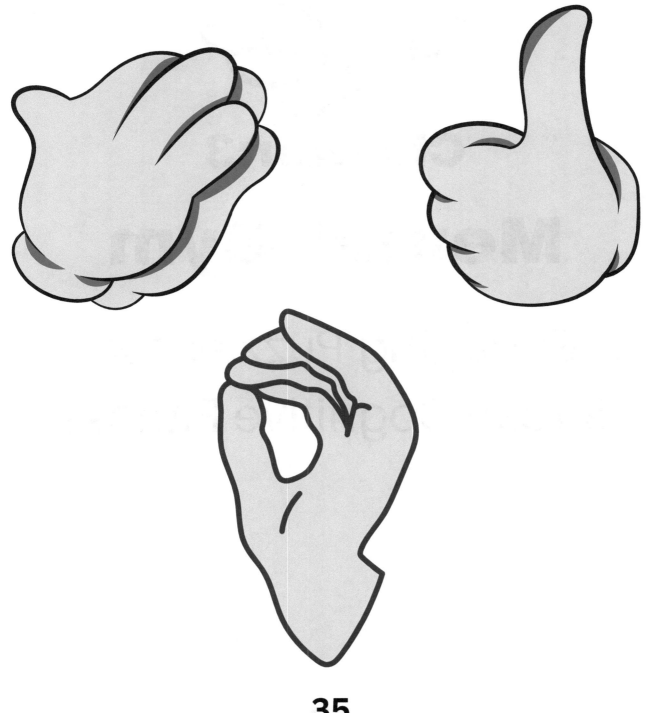

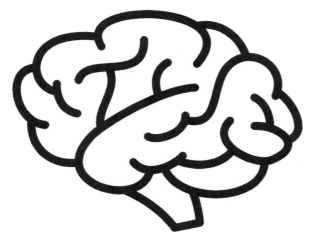

Chapter:3

Mental Gym

Engaging Puzzles for Stroke Cognitive Fitness

Word Search

Look for the words listed below.

```
P  C  U  P  A
U  S  S  A  E
N  H  U  T  W
D  A  N  L  U
R  T  K  R  Q
T  L  S  Z  O
```

Sun   Hat   Cup

37

Word Search

Circle the words given below.

```
L I P S W N
M D E N C H
O P N N C L
O S T A R A
N B O H W O
N C L O U D
```

lips   **cloud**

moon   **star**

38

Use the Number (1-3) to Complete the Sudoku .

Use each digit only once in each row, column and section.

1		3
	1	2
2		1

Use the Number (1-4) to Complete the Sudoku .

Use each digit only once in each row and column.

1	2		4
2		4	3
4	3	1	
	4	2	1

Word Scramble

Arrange the letters and correct the word.

M L E O N

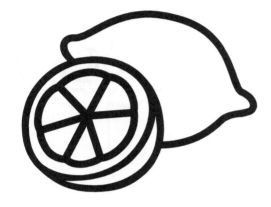

P P L E A

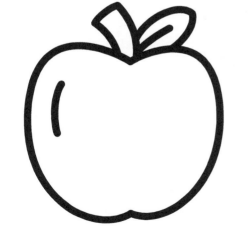

Word Scramble

Arrange the letters and Correct the words.

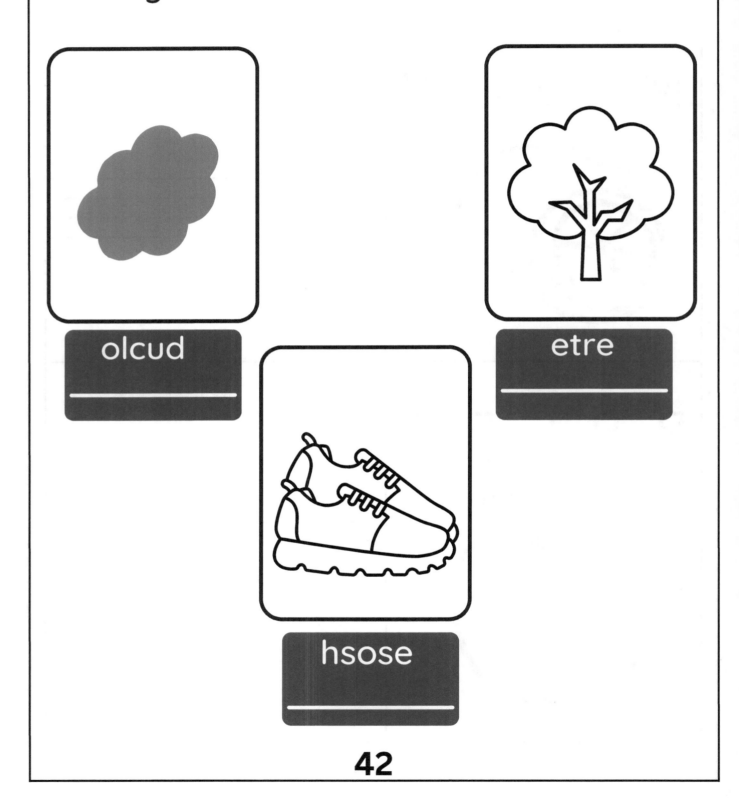

olcud
_____

etre
_____

hsose
_____

Lets Count the Shapes

Count and write your
answers in the chart below

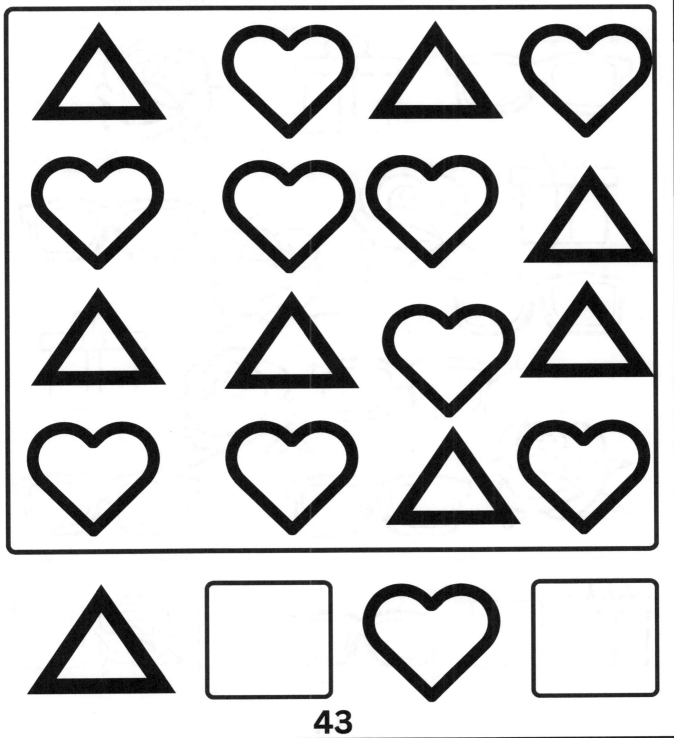

Lets Count the Objects

Count and write your answers in the boxes below

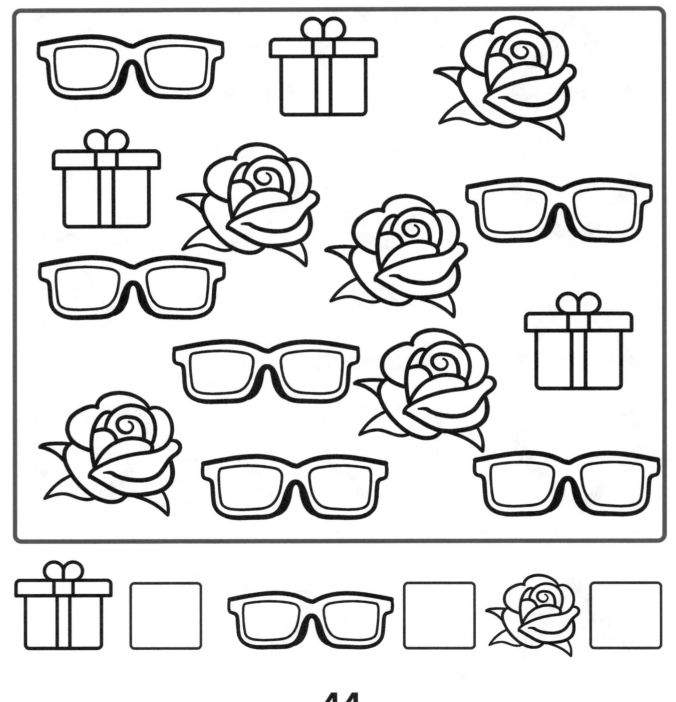

Vowel Activity

a e i o u

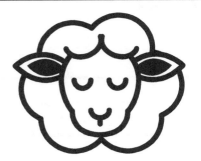

sh__p

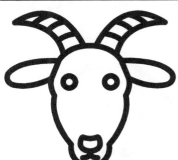

g___t

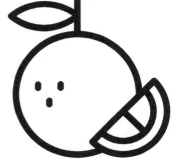

or_nge

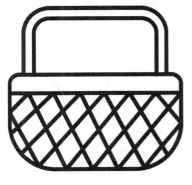

b_sket

fl_wer

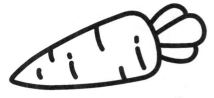

c_rr_t

Match and Write

Match the image with the first letter of the word.

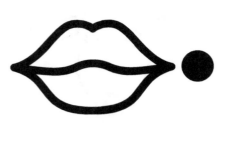 ● ●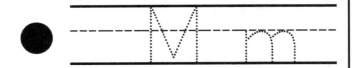

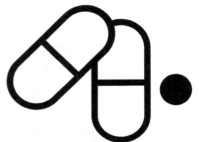 ● ●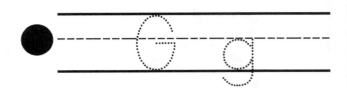

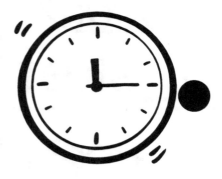 ● ●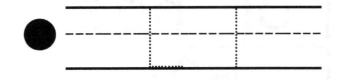

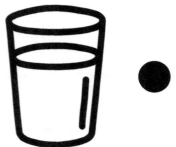 ● ●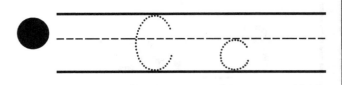

Word Formation

Connect the correct letter to build the word.

Picture	Letters	Answer
☀ (sun)	u s / n t	
🪲 (bug)	c u / B g	
🛖 (hut)	b H / t u	

Tell the Time in Hour.

Which clock is showing the correct time? Circle the correct one.

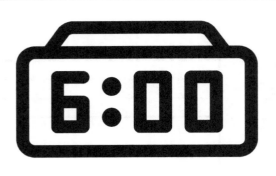

6:00

4:00

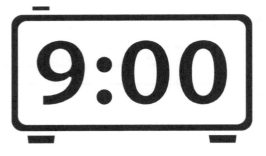

5:00

9:00

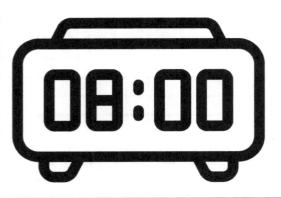

8:00

4:00

Connect the Dots

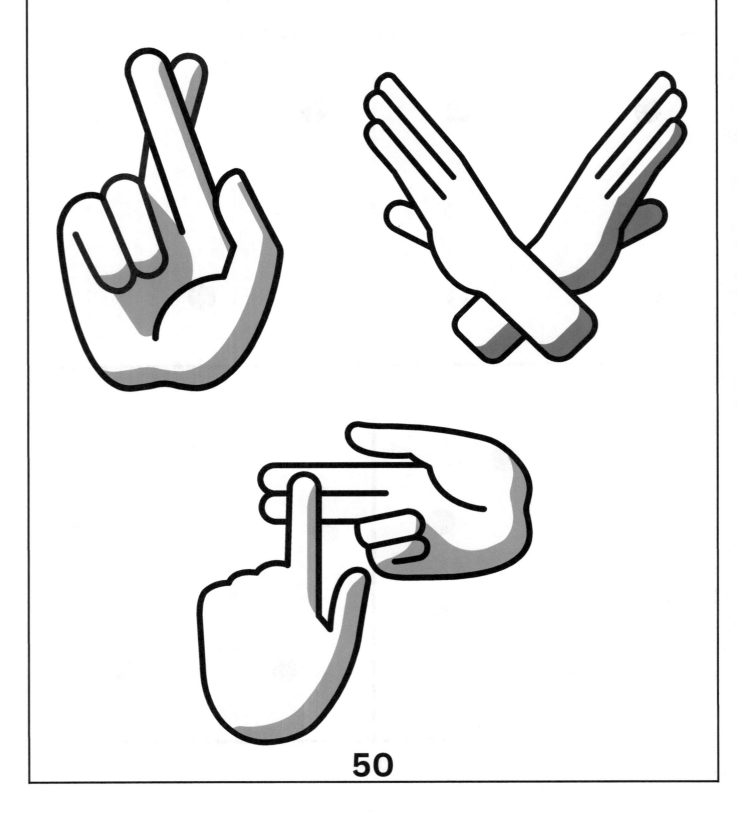

Time for Hand Movement

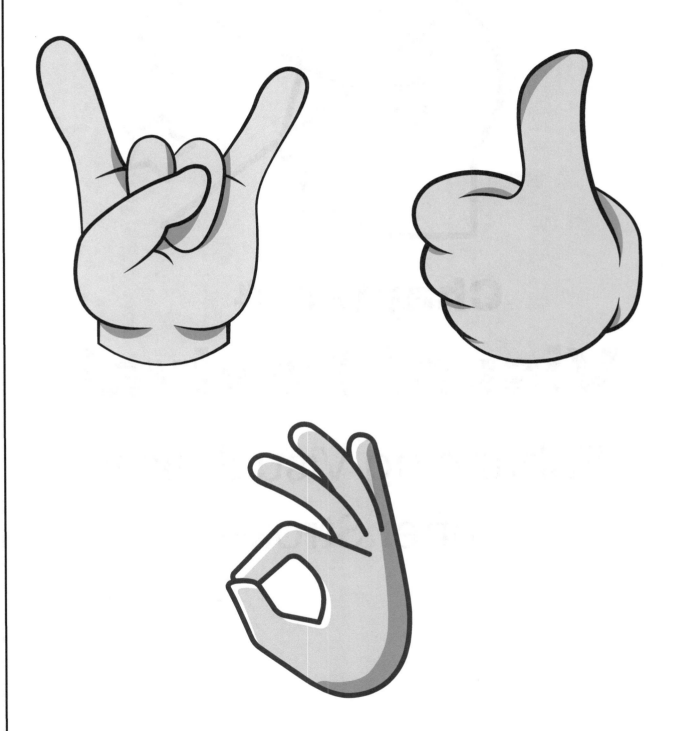

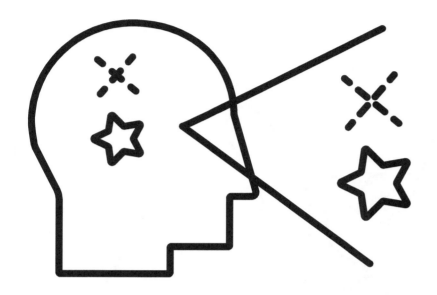

Chapter :4
Visual Revival

Enhancing Visual Skills
after Stroke

Arrange the Numbers from Smallest to largest

8   4   6   3   1

5   2   9   7   4

Match the Birds with their Shadows.

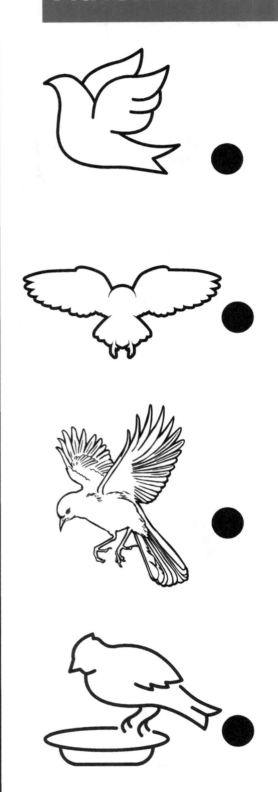
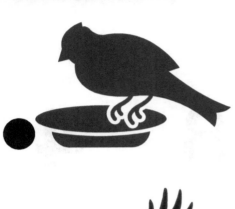
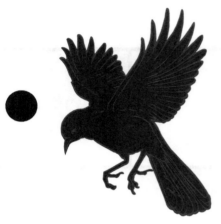

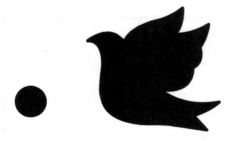

Count and Write the Number of Flowers in the Box Below.

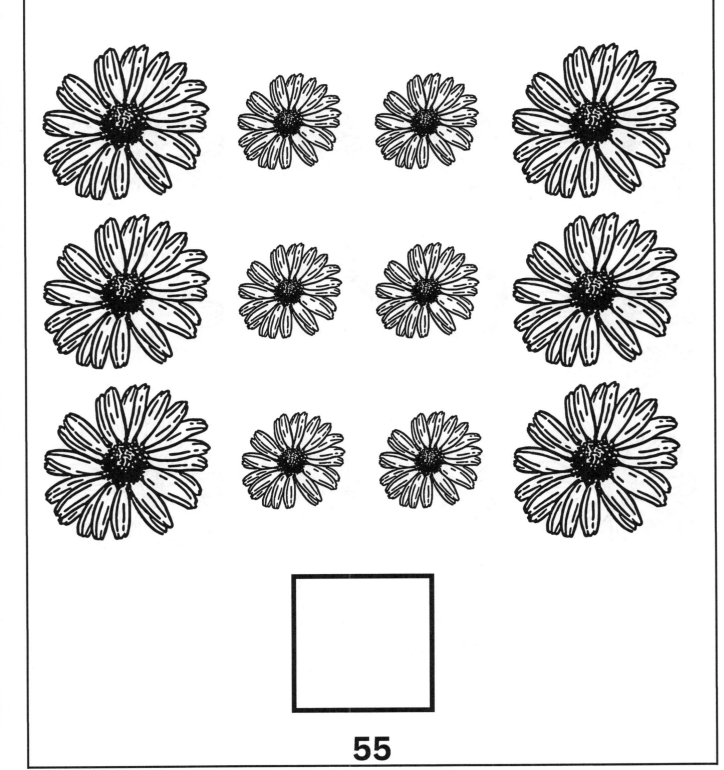

Color the Flower That has been Added.

Draw the Shapes from Smallest to Largest in the Chart Below.

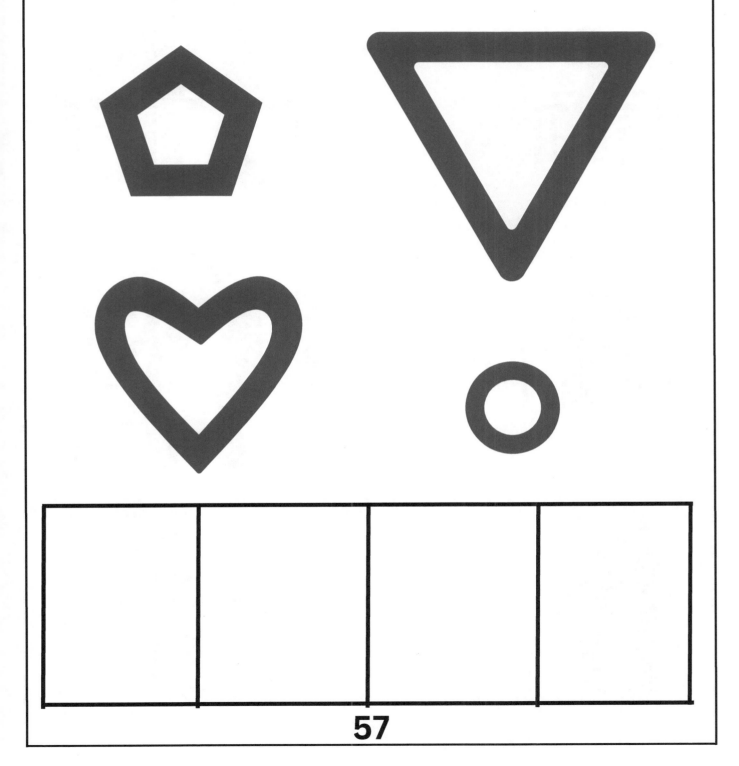

Find and Match each Small Images to its Large Image.

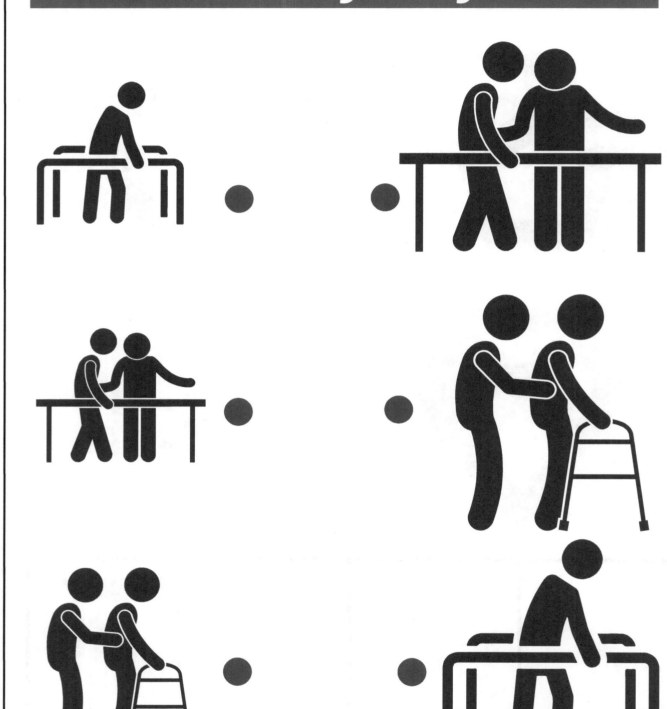

Circle the Things You Can Eat.

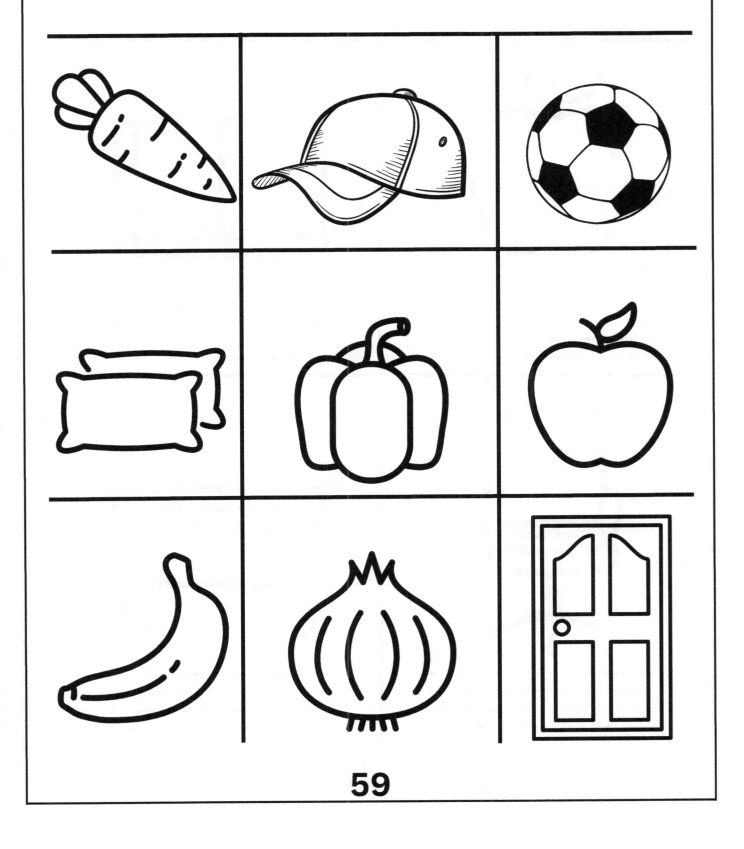

Write the Name of Each Object.

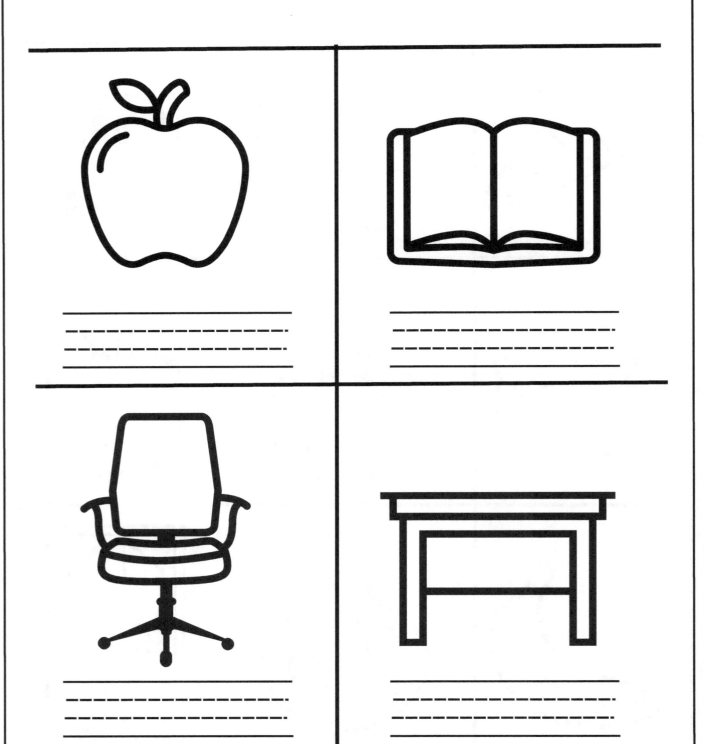

Identify and Circle Two Differences Between These Pictures

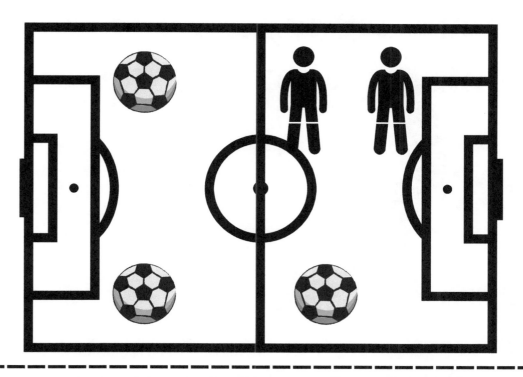

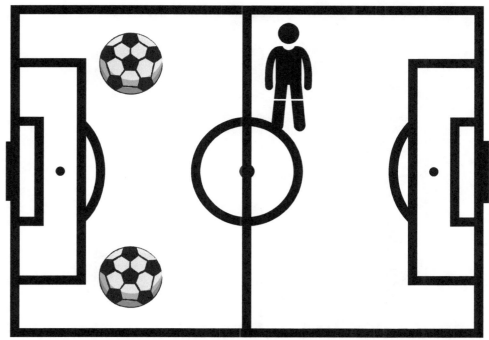

Draw the Other Half of Each Picture

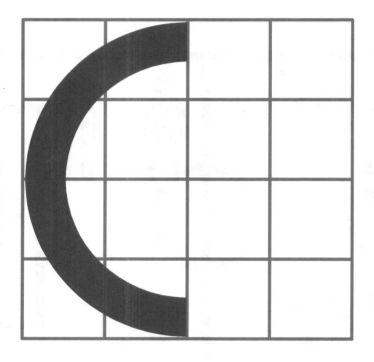

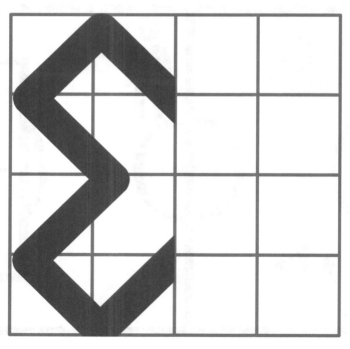

Color the Arrow Related to Their Direction.

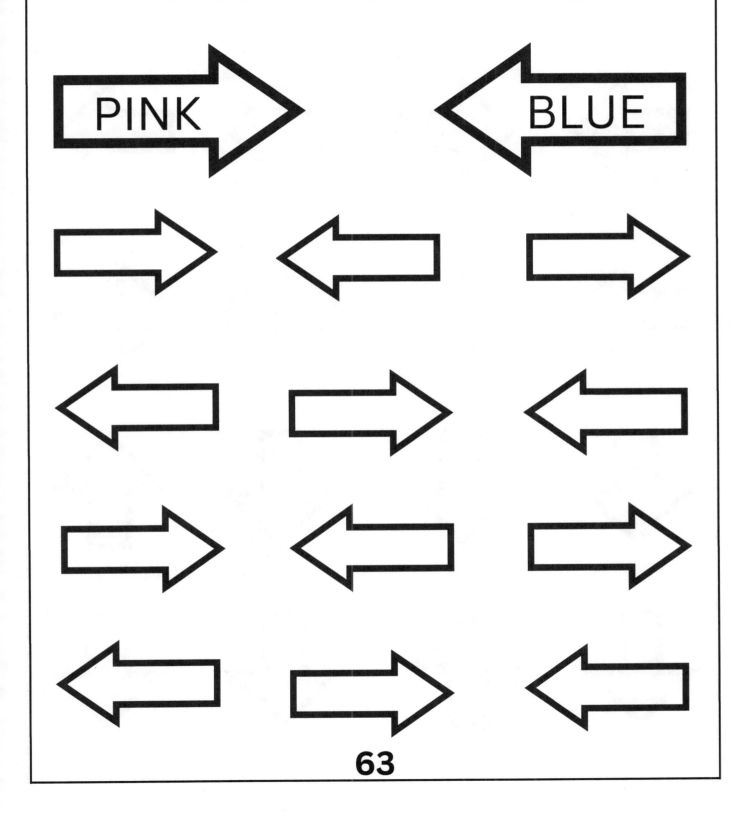

PINK

BLUE

Find Different in Each Group.

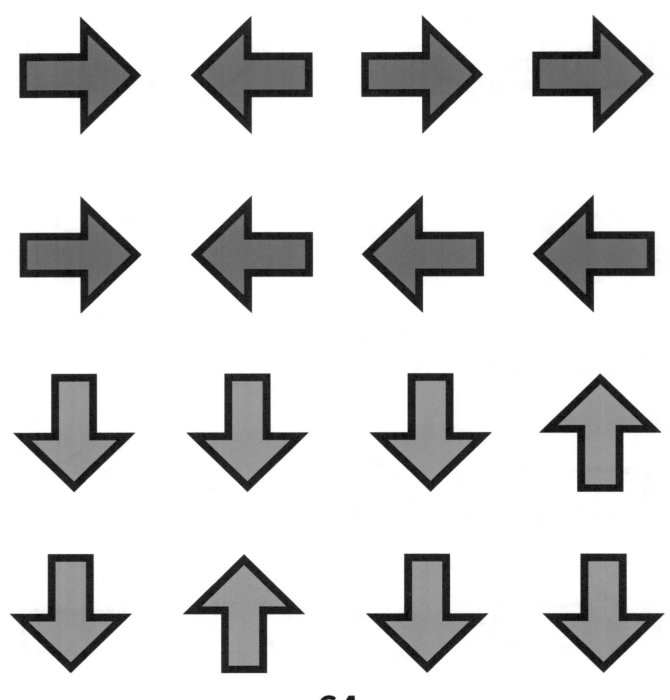

Guess the Emotions

Can you tell their emotions?
Choose from the words on the box.

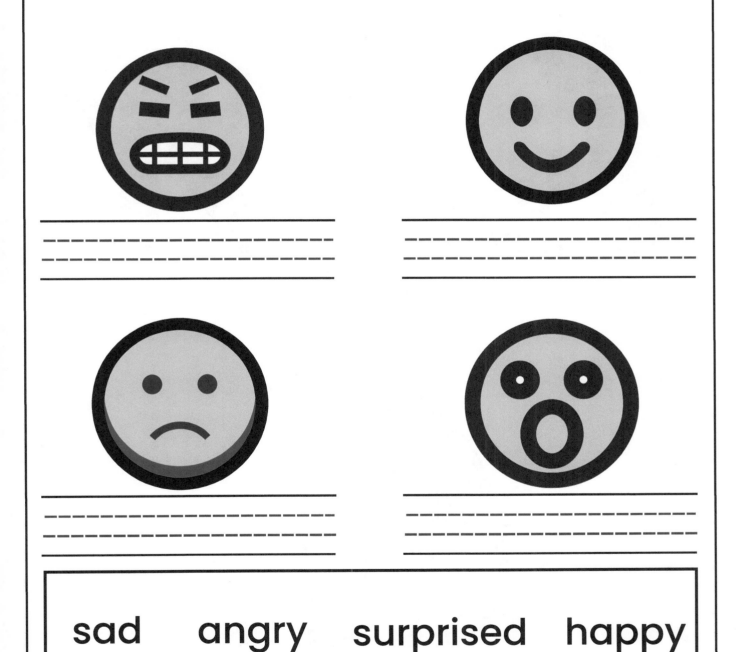

| sad | angry | surprised | happy |

Time for Legs Movement

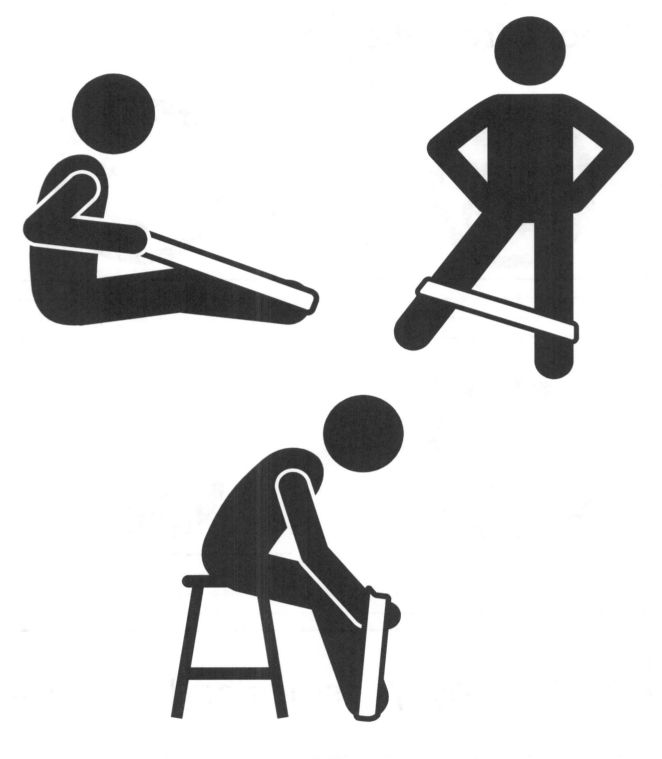

Time for Legs Movement

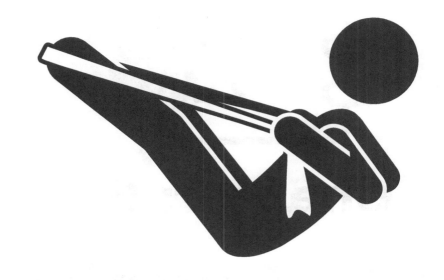

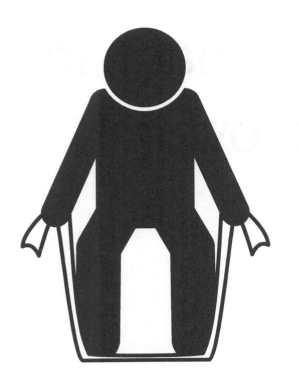

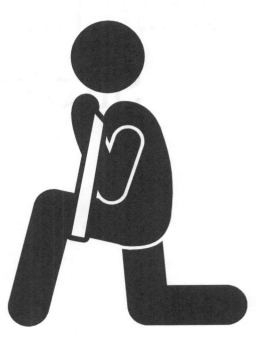

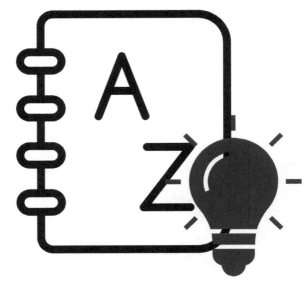

Chapter: 5

Words Regained

Mastering Language in Stroke Recovery

Sentence Making

Rearrange the words and make a correct sentence.

cup   The   full.   is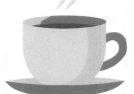

- -

day   The   hot.   is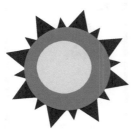

- -

pencil   is   short. The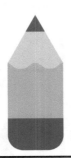

- -

Guess the Alphabet

Color all the boxes having alphabet "T" and find out the the letter.

T	T	T	T	T
Z	P	T	M	Y
B	X	T	F	U
D	O	T	N	G

Match the Rhymes

Pick a word from each group that rhymes with the other group and write below in the blanks.

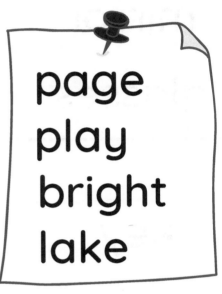

page
play
bright
lake

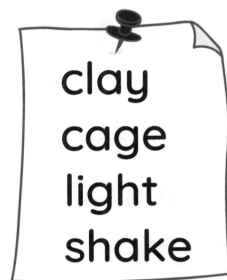

clay
cage
light
shake

- page and cage

- play and _ _ _ _

- bright and _ _ _ _ _

- lake and _ _ _ _ _

Identify the Picture

Color the box with the correct object name.

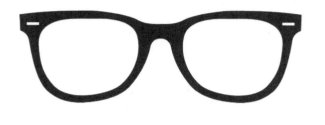

mirror

glasses

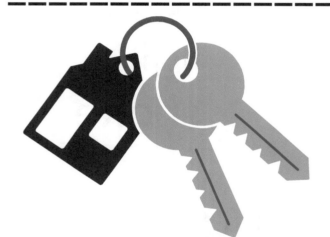

key

ring

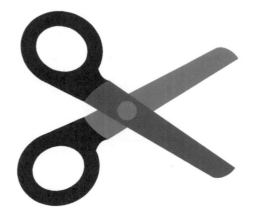

ruler

scissor

sentence completition

Use the correct word to complete the sentence.

- Frog can ＿＿＿＿＿ . (fly, jump)

- A ＿＿＿＿＿ makes honey. (bee, ant)

- Giraffes have ＿＿＿＿＿ necks. (long, short)

- The Earth is a ＿＿＿＿＿ . (planet, star)

- The Sun rises from ＿＿＿＿＿ . (East, West)

Places Identification

Put ✓ for Correct Sentence and ✗ for Wrong Sentences.

- She goes swimming in the pool.   ☐

- The Plane take off from the school.   ☐

- We deposit and withdraw money from bank.   ☐

- We get the medicine from police station.   ☐

- We can fill up our vehicles from gas station.   ☐

Match the Pictures.

Match the Column and complete the picture.

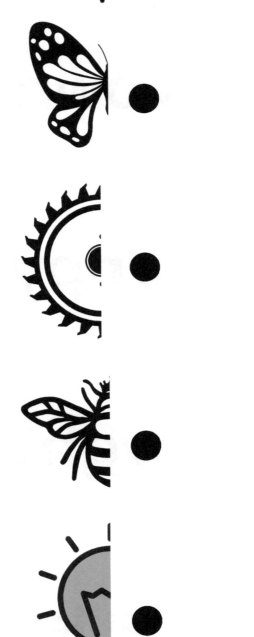

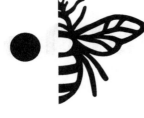

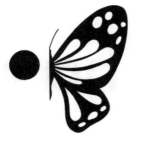

Try to match and make a word.

li •   • own

sm •   • ppy

cr •   • ght

ha •   • ile

Write the Missing Alphabets.

Each word has same double missing alphabets . Try to find out.

m _ _ n

b _ _ t

f _ _ l

ba _ _

fu _ _ y

a _ _ le

pu _ _ y

je _ _ y

77

Time for Legs Movement

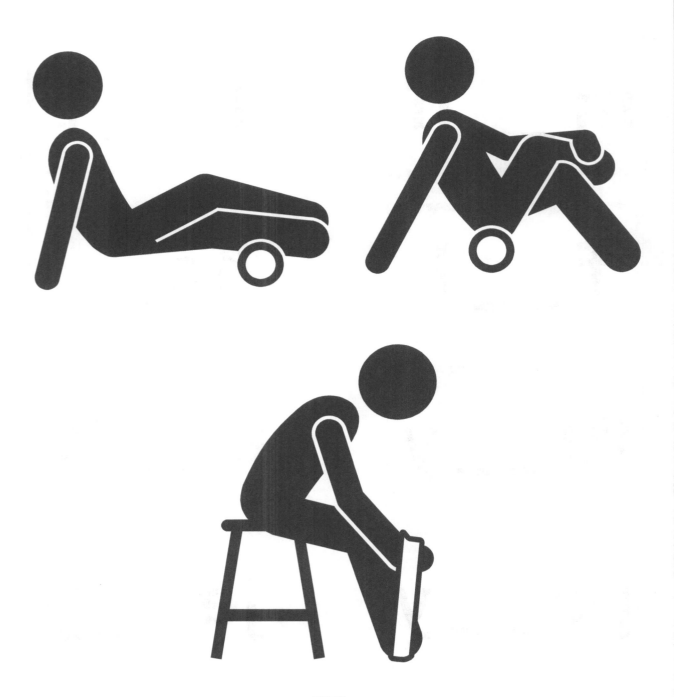

Time for Legs Movement

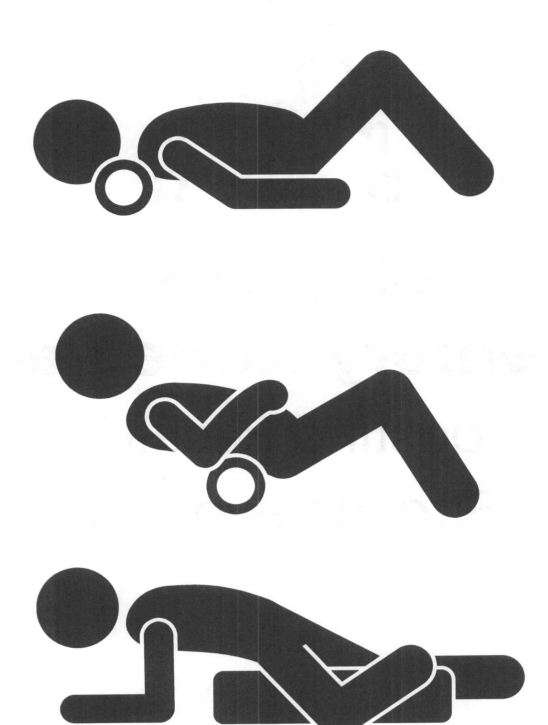

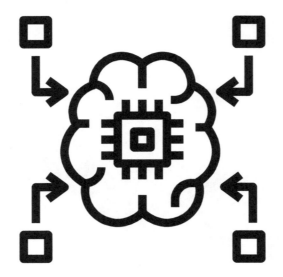

Chapter:6
Memory Renewed

Boosting Recall in
Stroke Recovery

Shape Recreation Pattern

Observe the pattern and memorize the place of each shape . On the next page draw shapes in the same location.

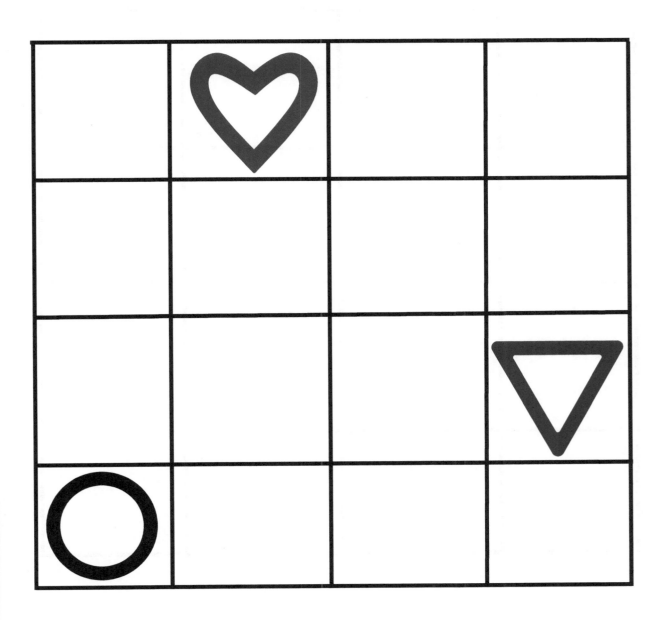

Shape Recreation Pattern

Remake the pattern that was presented on the previous page.

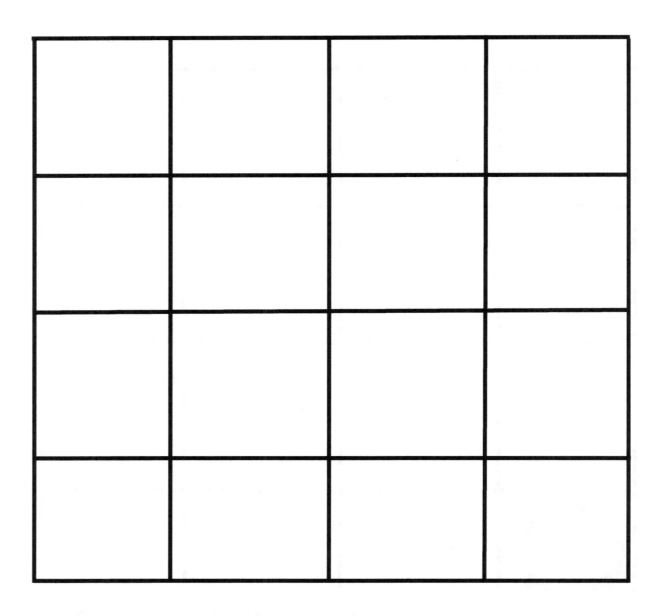

Recall your Relatives Names

Do you remember your father name ?

_____
- -
- -
_____

Do you remember you mother name?

_____
- -
- -
_____

Do you remember your date of birth?

_____
- -
- -
_____

Do you remember your city name?

_____
- -
- -
_____

Word Placement

Observe the pattern and memorize the place of each alphabet . On the next page write the alphabet in same pattern.

	A			S
		L		
				T
P				

Word Placement

Remake the word pattern that was presented on the previous page.

Identify the Object

Take a close look and remember the butterflies. On the next page circle new ones.

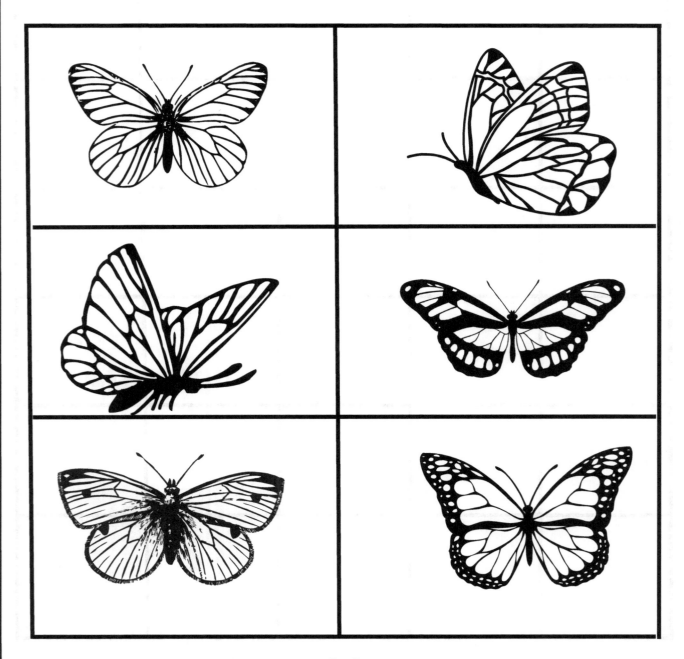

Identify the Object

Two butterflies has been added find out and circle them.

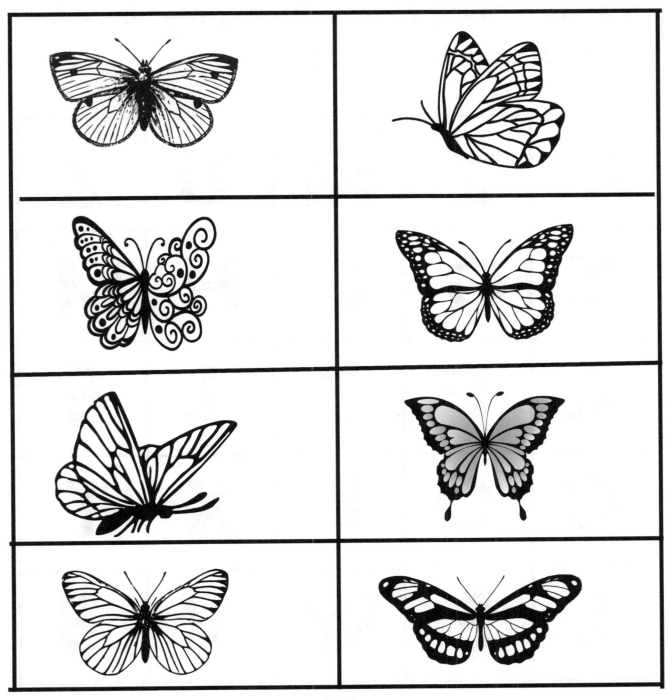

Connect the Alphabets

Connect the letters and find the word in the grid below.

Hint: Its a healthy fruit that comes in red, green or in yellow color.

X	Z	M	U	Z
Y	G	D	H	M
A	P	P	L	E
C	Q	E	X	T
L	F	W	V	B

Connect the Alphabets

Find the word in the grid below.

Hint: It's a color commonly related with nature and plant life.

A	G	U	H	P
Z	R	N	L	I
X	E	M	Y	S
W	E	T	C	E
B	N	R	Z	O

Letter Arrangement

Circle the six combinations that closely resemble the one in the rectangle.

uvmn

uvmn	ufmn	uvwn	uumn
vvmn	uvnn	uvmm	uvmn
uvcn	uvmn	uvpn	usmn
uvmm	uvsn	uvmn	uvtn
uvmn	urmn	udmn	uvqn
uvhn	uumn	uvmn	ulmn

Time for Legs Movement

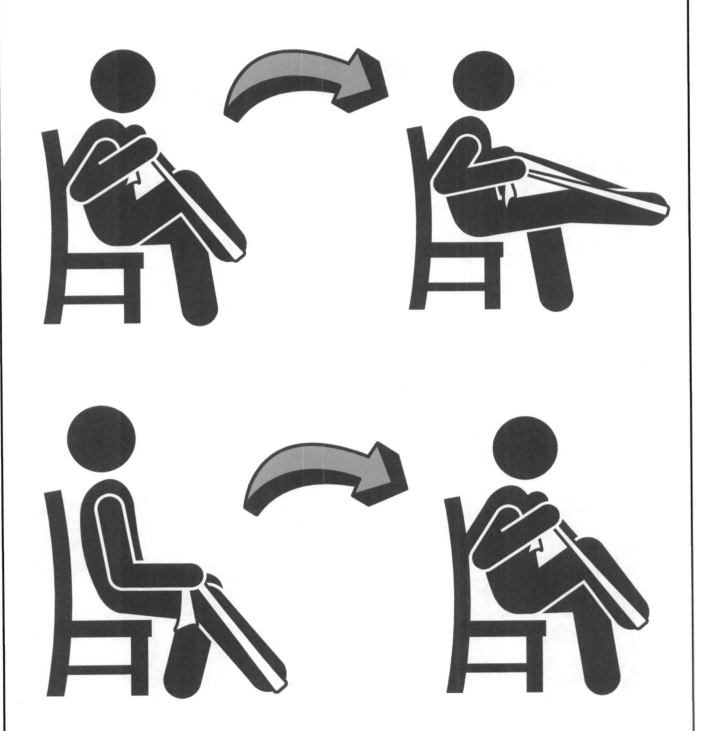

Time for Movement

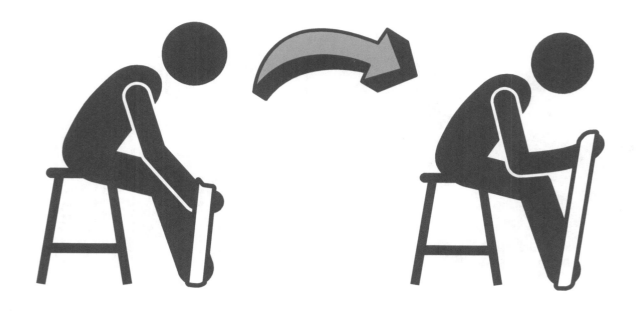

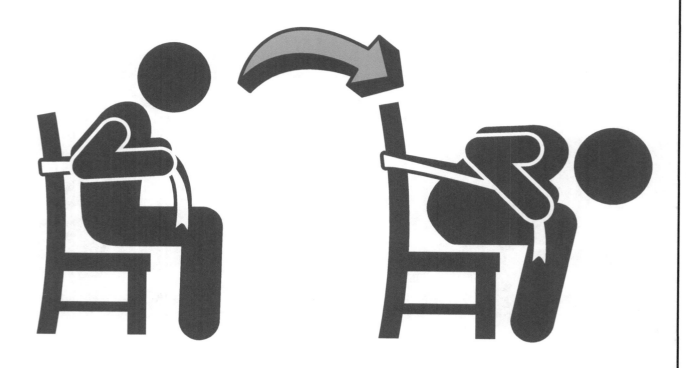

Solutions of Chapter 2

Circle the odd one

13   17   23

25   ⓒ   3

31   40   27

19   8   28

Circle the odd one

r   t   p   s

b   c   l   z

h   n   ⑤   u

x   t   p   y

Letter Hunt 🔍

Find all the letters 'x' and circle them.

Ⓧ   Ⓧ   Z   U

Ⓧ   T   M   Ⓧ

    Ⓧ

P   Ⓧ   W   N

S   Ⓧ   M   Ⓧ

Number Hunt 🔍

Find all the numbers 3 and circle them.

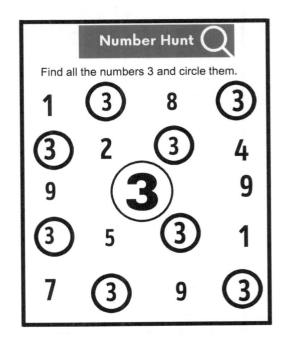

1   ③   8   ③

③   2   ③   4

9   ③   9

③   5   ③   1

7   ③   9   ③

Solutions of Chapter 3

Word Search

Look for the words listed below.

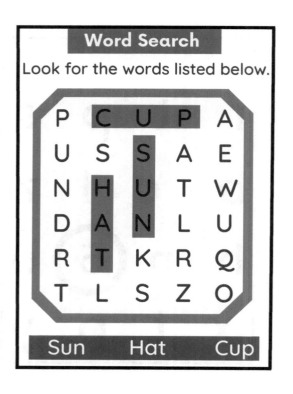

P	C	U	P	A
U	S	S	A	E
N	H	U	T	W
D	A	N	L	U
R	T	K	R	Q
T	L	S	Z	O

Sun   Hat   Cup

Word Search

Circle the words given below.

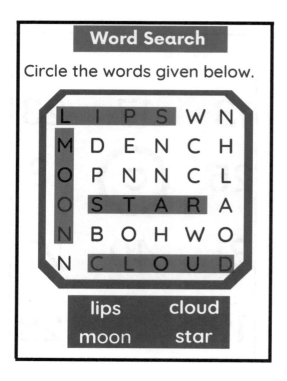

L	I	P	S	W	N
M	D	E	N	C	H
O	P	N	N	C	L
O	S	T	A	R	A
N	B	O	H	W	O
N	C	L	O	U	D

lips   cloud

moon   star

Use the Number (1-3) to Complete the Sudoku .

Use each digit only once in each row, column and section.

1	2	3
3	1	2
2	3	1

Use the Number (1-4) to Complete the Sudoku .

Use each digit only once in each row and column.

1	2	3	4
2	1	4	3
4	3	1	2
3	4	2	1

Solutions of Chapter 3

Word Scramble

Arrange the letters and Correct the words.

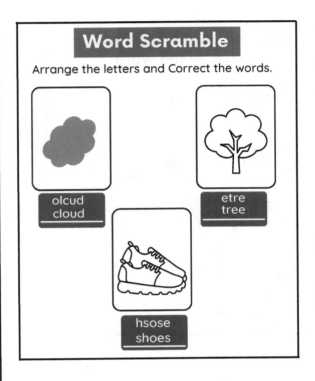

olcud
cloud

etre
tree

hsose
shoes

Lets count Shapes

Count and write your answers in the chart below

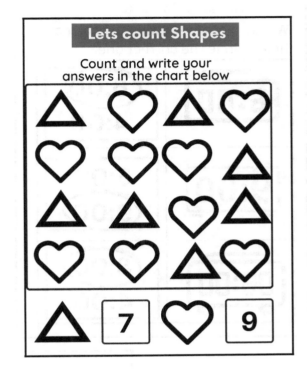

Counting Objects

Count and write your answers in the boxes below

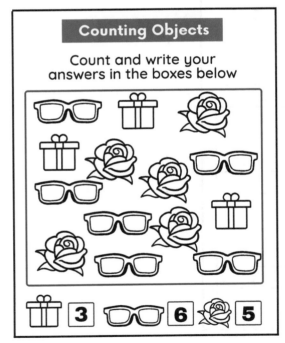

Vowel Activity

a e i o u

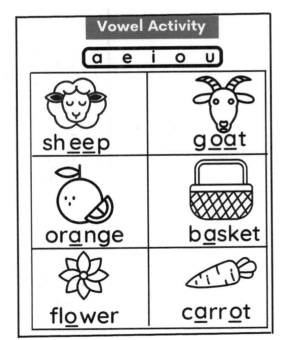

sh_ee_p

g_oa_t

or_a_nge

b_a_sket

fl_o_wer

c_a_rr_o_t

Solutions of Chapter 3

Tell the Time in Hour.

Which clock is showing the correct time? Circle the correct one.

6:00	(6:00) 4:00
9:00	5:00 (9:00)
08:00	(8:00) 4:00

Match and Write

Match the Image with the First Letter of the Word.

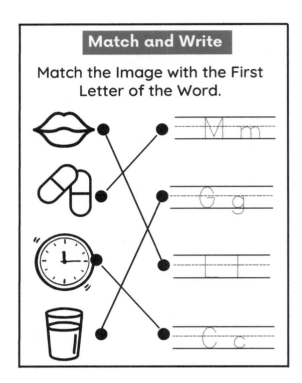

M m

G g

I i

C c

Word Formation

Connect the correct letter to build the word.

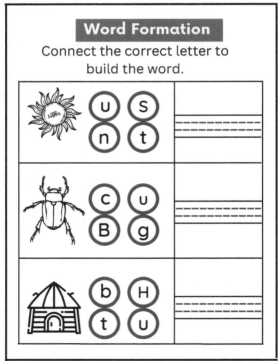

Arrange the Numbers from Smallest to largest

8 4 6 3 1

1	3	4	6	8

5 2 9 7 4

2	4	5	7	9

Match the birds with their shadows.

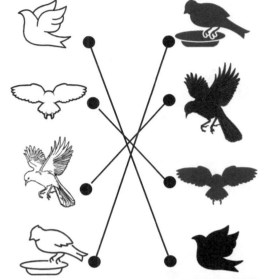

Count and Write the Number of Flowers in the Box Below.

12

Draw the Shapes from Smallest to Largest in the Chart Below.

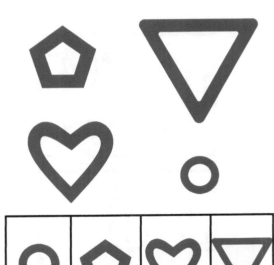

Solutions of Chapter 4

Find and Match each small images to its large image.

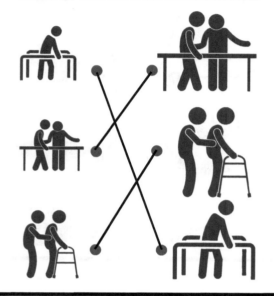

Circle the Things You Can Eat.

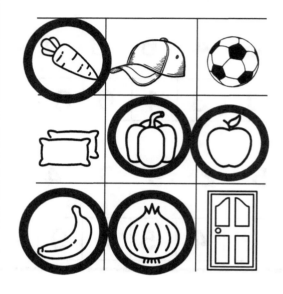

Identify and Circle Two Differences Between These Pictures

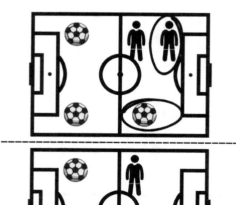

Find Different in Each Group.

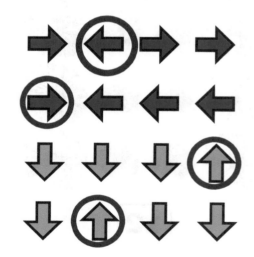

Solutions of Chapter 5

Sentence Making

Rearrange the words and make a sentence.

cup   The   full.   is

~~The   cup   is   full.~~

day   The   hot.   is

~~The   day   is   hot.~~

pencil   is   short.   The

~~The   pencil   is   short.~~

Guess the Alphabet

Color all the boxes having alphabet "T" and find out the the letter.

T	T	T	T	T
Z	P	T	M	Y
B	X	T	F	U
D	O	T	N	G

Answer is letter "T"

Match the Rhymes

Pick a word from each group that rhymes with the other group and write below in the blanks.

page
play
bright
lake

clay
cage
light
shake

- page and cage
- play and clay
- bright and light
- lake and shake

Identify the Picture

Color the box with the correct object name.

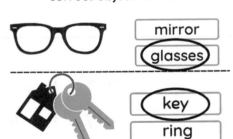

mirror
glasses

key
ring

 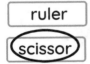

ruler
scissor

99

Solutions of Chapter 5

sentence completition

Use the correct word to complete the sentence.

- Frog can jump . (fly, jump)

- A bee makes honey. (bee, ant)

- Giraffes have long necks. (long, short)

- The Earth is a planet . (planet, star)

- The Sun rises from East . (East, West)

Places Identification

Put ✔ for Correct Sentence and ✖ for Wrong Sentences.

- She goes swimming in the pool. ✔

- The Plane take off from the school. ✖

- We deposit and withdraw money from bank. ✔

- We get the medicine from police station. ✖

- We can fill up our vehicles from gas station. ✔

Match the Pictures.

Match the Column and complete the picture.

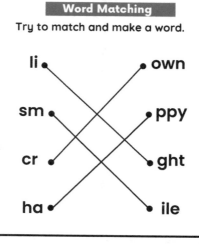

Word Matching

Try to match and make a word.

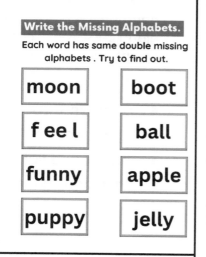

li — ile
sm — own
cr — ppy
ha — ght

Write the Missing Alphabets.

Each word has same double missing alphabets . Try to find out.

moon	boot
feel	ball
funny	apple
puppy	jelly

Identify the Object

Two butterflies has been added find out and circl them.

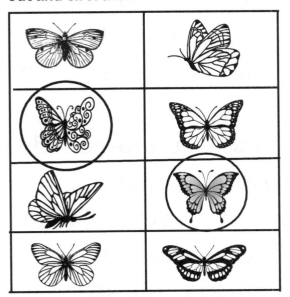

Connect the Alphabets

Connect the letters and find the word in the grid below.

Hint: Its a healthy fruit that comes in red, green or in yellow color.

X	Z	M	U	Z
Y	G	D	H	M
A	P	P	L	E
C	Q	E	X	T
L	F	W	V	B

Connect the Alphabets

Find the word in the grid below.

Hint: It's a color commonly related with nature and plant life.

A	G	U	H	P
Z	R	N	L	I
X	E	M	Y	S
W	E	T	C	E
B	N	R	Z	O

Letter Arrangement

Circle the six combinations that closely resemble the one in the rectangle.

uvmn

uvmn	ufmn	uvwn	uumn
vvmn	uvnn	uvmm	uvmn
uvcn	uvmn	uvpn	usmn
uvmm	uvsn	uvmn	uvtn
uvmn	urmn	udmn	uvqn
uvhn	uumn	uvmn	ulmn

Congratulations

Congratulations on completing the **"Stroke Recovery Activity Book"!**

Your dedication and commitment to your recovery journey have paid off. By finishing this book, you have not only acquired valuable knowledge and skills but also enhanced your cognitive abilities and physical capabilities.

Remember to practice and reinforce these newfound abilities regularly to maintain and further enhance your progress.This achievement is a testament to your resilience and unwavering spirit. We celebrate this significant milestone with you and wish you continued success and happiness in your ongoing recovery journey.

Help Janet Weasley grow by sending the reviews also share your solved activities. We will be thrilled to see that and your success is a reminder for other stoke patients that with dedication and the right resources, stroke recovery is possible.

**Warmest congratulations,
Janet Weasley**

Explore our wide range of good selling activity books crafted specifically for adults and seniors to relax the mind and soul.

www.amazon.com
https://www.amazon.com/dp/B0BVDF14ZY
Amazon ASIN:B0BVDF14ZY

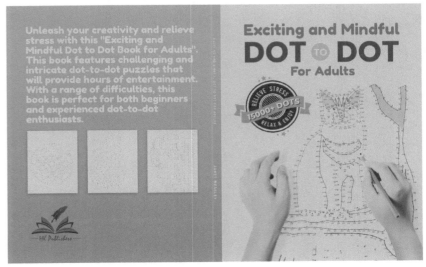

www.amazon.com
https://www.amazon.com/dp/B0C47Q563W
Amazon ASIN:B0C47Q563W

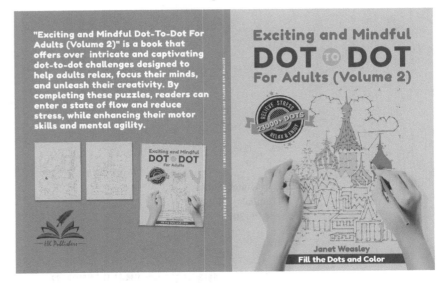

19477984R00060